The Psychology Behind Weight Loss

The Role of Mindset
In Weight Loss Success

Ron Kness

Published by:

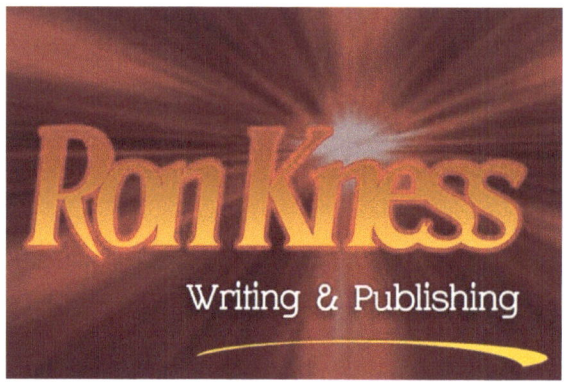

https://ronknesswriting.com

Ron Kness

San Tan Valley, AZ

United States of America

ISBN: 9781070768380

Sneak Peek

What you "think" is more important than what you "do" when it comes to achieving and maintaining a healthy weight.

Your brain can quickly begin delivering the weight loss results you have longed for when you do *one thing first*.

Odds are, no matter who you are, how old you are, whether you are a man, woman or child, you need to lose some excess fat and body weight to become healthier and happier.

Here's why I know I can make that broad statement.

- The National Health and Nutrition Examination Survey says that 2 in every 3 adults is either overweight or obese.
- 1 in 3 adults are obese.
- 1 in 6 children and adolescents are obese, and 3 out of every 5 are overweight.
- The one, simple thing you need to do before you follow any weight loss advice is …

Change your mindset and break through psychological blocks

Don't believe the lie that change is slow. The minute you decide that you are going to develop a mindset that leads to health and well-being through weight loss, that mental change is instant.

Then, you must take action on your new mindset. The problem is that most people don't understand what that means or the mental obstacles that keep them from lasting weight loss success.

Most people don't know the step-by-step process that needs to be followed to program their brain for weight loss success.

If you have tried miracle diets, exercise, medicine and everything under the sun to lose weight and you have failed, we have some good news to share with you today ...

You can finally discover how to lose unwanted weight and keep it off. My book ***The Psychology Behind Weight Loss - The Role of Mindset In Weight Loss Success*** shows you how.

Legal/Disclaimer Notices

Disclaimer Notice:

Please note the information contained within this document is for educational and entertainment purposes only and is not intended as medical advice. Medical advice should always be obtained from a qualified medical professional for any health conditions or symptoms associated with them.

Every attempt has been made to provide accurate, up to date and reliable complete information. No warranties of any kind are expressed or implied. Readers acknowledge that the author is not engaging in the rendering of legal, financial, medical or professional advice.

By reading this document, the reader agrees that under no circumstances are we responsible for any losses, direct or indirect, which are incurred as a result of the use of information contained within this document, including, but not limited to, —errors, omissions, or inaccuracies.

See your healthcare professional before starting any diet, health or exercise program!

Table of Contents

The Psychology Behind Weight Loss

A lot of people struggle with weight. According to Health Data, some 160 million Americans are overweight or obese. According to the Centers For Disease Control, 2/3rds of American adults are overweight or obese.

Weight loss is a struggle for thousands, and even when they manage to lose weight, keeping it off proves to be a challenge. Most people believe that to lose weight, all you need to focus on is eating less and exercising more. And from a physiological standpoint, it is true; you must burn more calories than you take in to lose weight.

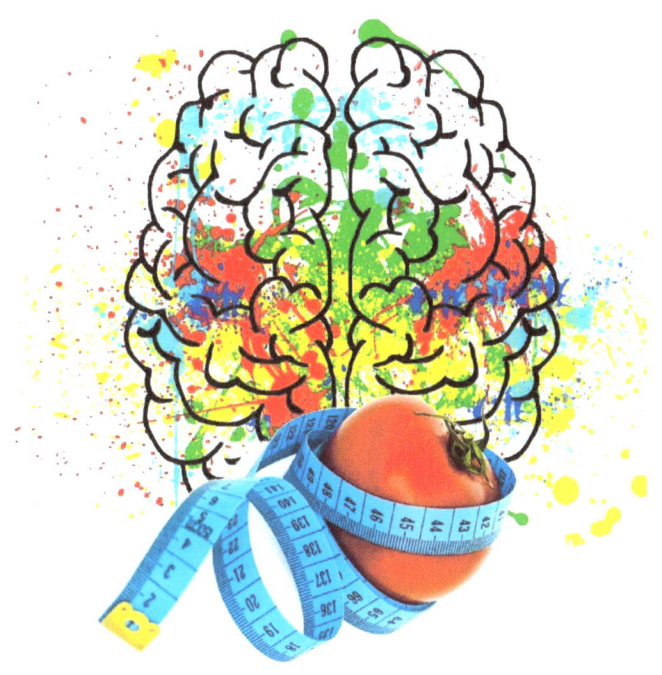

But, unfortunately, it's just not that simple. To effectively lose weight, you must change various aspects of your mindset, beliefs, and bad habits related to food and exercise that landed you where you are today.

In fact, psychology is 99% of weight loss.

If you want to lose weight and keep it off, you must deal with the emotions, beliefs, and psychological baggage you carry around about yourself, food, weight, body image, and eating.

If you want to become healthier and, in the process lose weight, then you need to change how you think of the process. You don't need to diet; you need to shift your mindset. You don't need fewer calories; you need fewer negative thoughts and critical self-talk. In short, you need to understand how it's your mind, not your stomach, that control what, when, and how you eat.

According to the American Council On Exercise, *"with the proper mindset, nearly any weight-loss program can be effective. Unfortunately, the unifying trait of the more than 65 percent of dieters who regain weight within the first year and the 85 percent of dieters who regain weight within three years is an unhealthy, self-sabotaging psychological mindset. That means that most dieters do not know how to think like a thin person and are instead filled with irrational self-talk that serves as hindrances to effective lifestyle change."*

We have examined all the reasons why losing weight is a difficult process, including the many ways your mind plays tricks or derails your efforts time and again. After we've explored the psychology of weight loss, we'll examine practical and tested strategies for how to change your mind, so that you can improve your health. If you are ready to begin your weight loss journey, then it's time to start by examining your mind.

Why Weight Loss Is So Hard

The reasons weight loss is difficult has very little to do with your genetics, your chronic illnesses, or your bone structure, in spite of what we all tell ourselves. It is hard because of one simple fact: Eating is not just something you do to stay alive. Eating is a profoundly emotional experience that comes attached to a whole host of memories, biases, and needs that have nothing to do with nutrition.

The first step to eating healthier and losing weight is to understand how your mind is controlling your choices about food. Once you pull back the curtain and see how subtle and not-so-subtle patterns of thinking control your preferences, you can begin to make changes that will, over time, help you develop the healthy habits you desire. ***Because losing weight isn't about changing your life for right now, it's about changing your life for good.*** Here's why that tends to be harder than we'd like.

Your Choices and Habits Say a Lot About Your Needs

If you want to understand your real emotions and preferences when it comes to food, then you need to start by examining your patterns and behaviors. To really understand why eating, dieting, and body images are such issues for you, you must get into the details of what and how you eat. It is here that you will discover what you need to know about what really needs to change in your life.

Any time that you are finding happiness, nurturing, peace, or some other emotion from eating, then it is necessary to examine why you aren't getting those emotions from other, non-food experiences in your life. If eating chocolate helps you relax and feel in control, then you have identified a need that you are filling using food that could be filled in other ways. If you tend to overeat at night, are you feeling lonely? Or bored? Or anxious?

Try this exercise. Think of one of the most favorite things you enjoy eating. Think about the experience of eating it, of enjoying it. What feelings come to mind as you think about eating this food? What images pop into your head? Pay attention to all the things that bubble up in your mind as you sit and think about eating this food.

Now, what can you learn from this? What emotional needs are you getting from eating this food, and is it possible you could get the same emotional benefits from other, healthier non-food sources in your life? What other ways of living could you embrace that allow you to experience the same positive emotions while also making healthier choices for yourself – food or otherwise?

Dieting Won't Make Your Inner Critic Go Away

Most people get to a point where they want to lose weight because they wish they felt better about themselves. They are tired of listening to the inner critic that is always telling them of their failings and poor choices. But what most of us don't realize is this:

That inner critic, that voice that's always telling you what you did wrong or how you messed up? It doesn't have to talk about food or your weight. The root of that voice runs way deeper than your size or what you eat.

The inner critical voice you are hearing is the symptom of a fundamental critical negative attitude you have about yourself. Even if you lose all the weight you want to lose, that voice will resurface with a new focus. If you're going to win the battle of the bulge for good, then what you really need to do is silence that negative inner critic and learn to love yourself positively for exactly who you are.

Start by listening carefully to that inner critic. What things is it criticizing you for? How long has this voice been around, and where do you think it comes from? When was the first time you criticized yourself? How would you like to treat yourself instead? What can you say to this inner critic to explain how it is making you feel?

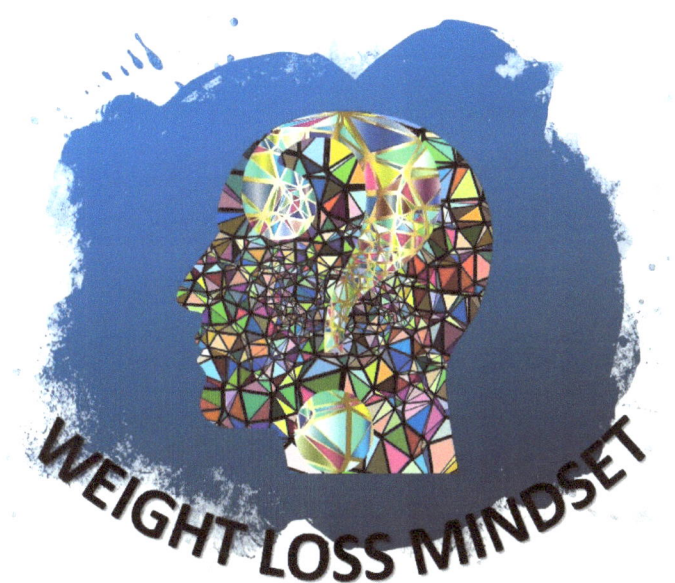

Next, make a commitment to stop shaming yourself for setbacks in your behaviors. Have it out with that critical inner voice. It's time to embrace more positive self-love and personal power and say "no" to this voice that is controlling your life. Start by looking in the mirror and saying the words out loud that this inner voice is saying in your head. Voicing these words makes it clear just how wounding they are. How do these words make you feel? Then, fight back.

Respond to that inner voice with all the reasons why you are still worthy of happiness and love, regardless of your size. Embrace your personal power to love and accept yourself and show that little voice who's boss. Look deeply at all the ways that voice is guiding you to make poor choices or unhealthy decisions in your life.

It's About Your Relationship With Yourself

Most of the time, weight loss efforts are challenged when our bodies don't match our desired sense of self. But this is actually the opposite of how you should be thinking. Instead of changing your weight or size, it's necessary to change how you feel about yourself.

Once you learn more self-love and less self-loathing, you'll be able to develop new, healthier habits for the right reasons, which is because you want to be happy and enjoy a long, healthy life.

Learning to love yourself is hard work. But with it comes a genuine acceptance of yourself for all your strengths and weaknesses and a knowledge that, any changes you make are to build your strengths, not to change who you are or overcome your faults.

Positive self-love is vital to true and lasting weight loss because, when you love yourself, you are making decisions and developing new habits for the right reasons.

It's Not About The Diet Plan

Most people who are attempting to lose weight have tried to diet before. And even if you were successful at losing weight in the past, the odds say that you have likely gained back some or all (or more) of what you lost before. This is especially true if you have used any type of "diet" program to lose weight. Diets, quite simply, don't work; healthy eating plans as part of a healthy lifestyle do work and they work well.

You didn't get fat overnight. You got there for years of everyday, unhealthy choices. You got there by habit. If you want to get "un-fat," you need to do it the same way — years of everyday, healthy choices, of better practices.

And yet, we spend billions of dollars every year chasing the next diet fad guaranteed to help you lost ten pounds fast. But the second you start eating in your old ways again, because most diets don't teach you how to eat once off of the diet, it is no surprise that the weight comes right back. Because you didn't change your habits. You changed your diet for a short time.

Instead of thinking about dieting, think about health. Instead of thinking about what you can't eat, think about what fuel your body needs. Instead of looking at eating as an emotional experience, look at it as a functional one.

Think about someone you know who has successfully quit a bad habit (like smoking). What did they have to do? And do they still have to work at it every day? Losing weight for good requires a commitment to healthy choices every day - for the rest of your life! Not for the next 30-day challenge. Not until you shed those extra pounds. Every.. day.. Forever!

Weight Loss Psychology: Your Brain May Be Holding You Back

Why is it that millions of people struggle to lose weight and keep it off? Jim Keller, Obesity Psychologist and Director of Behavioral Health at the WeightWise Bariatric Program in Oklahoma City believes that weight loss is a challenge because the body and brain are designed to eat.

Keller asserts that the causes of obesity are complex and composed of an intricate and complicated matrix of genetic, biological and environmental factors.

"Shifting your mindset about how to lose weight is the biggest factor in losing weight," says NYC-based therapist Kathryn Smerling. *"We can't shift our weight from the outside without realizing the correct inner resolve and intention."*

Change is difficult, but what is extremely helpful is gaining insight into the process of changing behavior.

According to Dr. Howard Rankin, behavioral change expert, *"for better or worse, our core, emotional values will ultimately determine our choices. Once we identify our heartfelt desires, we can use them to create a healthy lifestyle that reflects our best self. Our deepest values can be summoned to keep us on track, especially when we are facing temptations and distractions. They can also serve as our compass when we go astray"* (https://www.huffpost.com/entry/weight-loss-psychology_n_881706).

Psychological Blocks To Weight Loss

Why is it that we cannot just make a decision to lose weight, do it and keep it off? The answer to that question is complicated and many factors play a role, most of which are psychological in nature.

Lack Of Self-Awareness

Self-awareness is always the first step to change of any kind. In order to make changes, you must identify *and* accept what psychological blocks exist within you in your weight loss efforts. Once you know what they are, you can address them and facilitate change. Knowledge, journaling, workbooks and a coach or therapist can all help you to gain that awareness you need.

Self-Sabotage

Do you believe that you deserve to be fit, healthy and at a normal weight? Many people don't. This psychological block is very real and deters your success quickly and mercilessly.

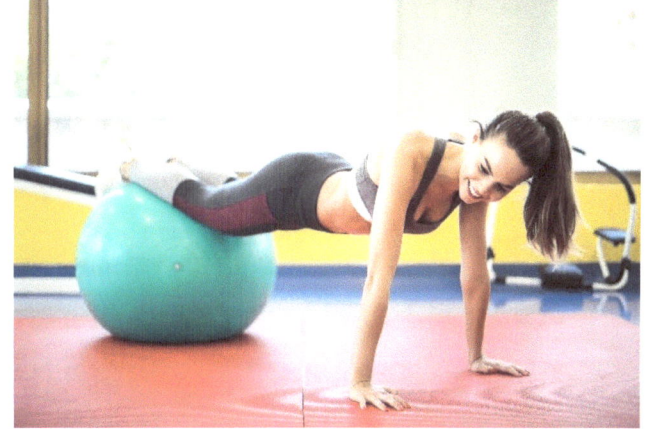

Where there is low self-esteem or worse yet, self-hatred issues, staying overweight and being overweight can be a subconscious form of self-punishment. When you don't believe you deserve it, or you have a need to punish yourself, self-sabotage will rear its ugly head quickly stopping long-term success in its tracks. These can be deep-seeded issues, and a licensed mental health professional can help you work through them.

Your Thoughts And Beliefs Play A Key Role In Self-Sabotage

Consider this scenario: You're at dinner and see cheesecake on the menu. You think, "it's only cheesecake, I had a long day, my body is craving it so it must need it, or I went to the gym today, a little piece won't hurt me." You eat the cheesecake, then you feel guilty and anxious and berate yourself for falling into the same old trap.

The initial thought or thoughts is what led to giving into that cheesecake, other examples of such thoughts include:

- Why should I suffer, I am starving
- I've had a long hard day, I deserve it
- It's okay to cheat tonight, I will start over tomorrow
- What's the point, I have no willpower anyway
- I have no control over my cravings, it's too hard to fight them
- I will eat this but workout for 2 hours tomorrow to make up for it
- I shouldn't deprive myself

You must change your thought patterns in order to strengthen your resistance and replace negative self-sabotaging thoughts with positive empowering accurate and rational thoughts.

Why should I suffer, I am starving – *instead: it's uncomfortable but it will go away"*

I've had a long hard day, I deserve it – *instead: "I deserve the best health and body"*

It's okay to cheat tonight, I will start over tomorrow – *instead: "tomorrow is today, there are no more excuses"*

What's the point, I have no willpower anyway – *instead: "I have total control over my actions and what I eat"*

I have no control over my cravings, it's too hard to fight them – *instead: "I have a craving, but that doesn't mean I have to give in, it will pass"*

I will eat this but workout for 2 hours tomorrow to make up for it – *instead: "I won't eat this because I am committed to my own good health and weight loss"*

I shouldn't deprive myself – *instead: "I deprive myself of what is unhealthy, but with that I am giving myself so much more that is"*

Your Emotional Readiness

Being unprepared for the changes to come is a major psychological block to weight loss. Preparing yourself both emotionally and mentally for change is key. Often, dieters view dieting as some temporary event, and when the diet is over, they simply return to business as usual. This is a mistake, as it rarely results in any lasting weight loss success.

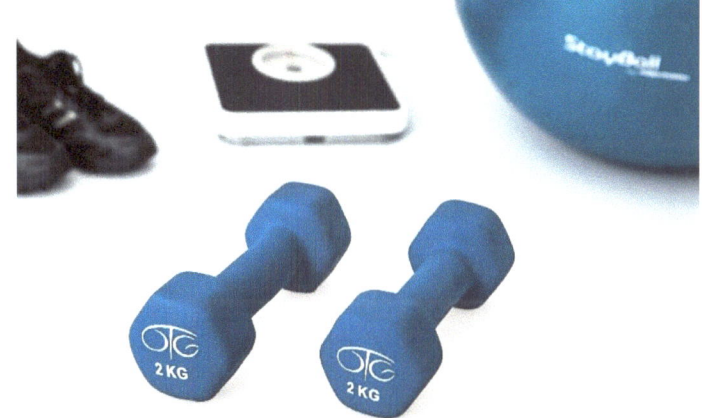

Lasting weight loss requires a major shift in mindset, habits and behaviors and this requires an earnest effort in preparing yourself for change, *a major change.*

Distorted Thinking

The most egregious cognitive distortion that blocks people from losing weight is..."I should be able to eat anything I want, whenever I want." Unfortunately, this is a pipe dream.

In order to have the proper mindset and the correct psychology for weight loss, you must change your thought process towards a healthier lifestyle, this includes:

- Learning to feel satisfied with just being full after a meal, but not stuffed
- Learning to identify real hunger versus a mental desire to eat for other reasons
- Being able to control cravings
- The ability to monitor food intake – which includes mindful eating and portion control
- Develop healthy coping skills for stress and negative emotions
- Be comfortable with and accept that food restrictions and portion sizes are a natural part of a healthy weight
- Accept that lasting habit changes are needed for lasting weight loss and this means that healthy thinking must be maintained for life

Poor Self-Esteem

One of the biggest blocks to weight loss is poor self-esteem. Poor self-esteem is likely a huge contributing factor to you being overweight and it is also one of the main blocks to losing the weight and keeping it off. If you don't feel that you deserve to be healthy, then it is difficult to do what you need to get there.

It's as simple as this - when you love yourself, you want to take care of yourself, and do the best for yourself, and being overweight or obese does not comply with those needs. In fact, it can be viewed as a form of self-abuse.

There is also the fact that for those with low self-esteem or worse yet, self-hatred issues, being and staying overweight can be a subconscious form of self-punishment. These can be deep seeded issues, and a licensed mental health professional can help you work through them.

Emotional Distortion: Connecting Food To Feelings

How many times has the thought of a cheeseburger and fries (or whatever) made you happy, elated, alleviated your stress or improved your day? This association of food with feelings and using food as an emotional crutch is an unhealthy thought process and a very real psychological block to weight loss and healthy eating.

Living To Eat Versus Eating To Live

Notice the difference between the two mentalities. "Eating to live" is a healthy mindset that considers food as sustenance and a requirement for survival. On the other hand, the "living to eat" mindset is obsessed with food and uses food as an emotional crutch, and typically results in eating for reasons other than hunger.

Until you shift your mindset towards "eating to live," and seeing food as it was intended for sustenance, it will be difficult to lose weight and most importantly to keep it off, as your food obsession will take over all your dietary decisions.

Body Shame

Syracuse University research found that *"the more dissatisfied women are with their bodies, the more likely they are to avoid exercise."*

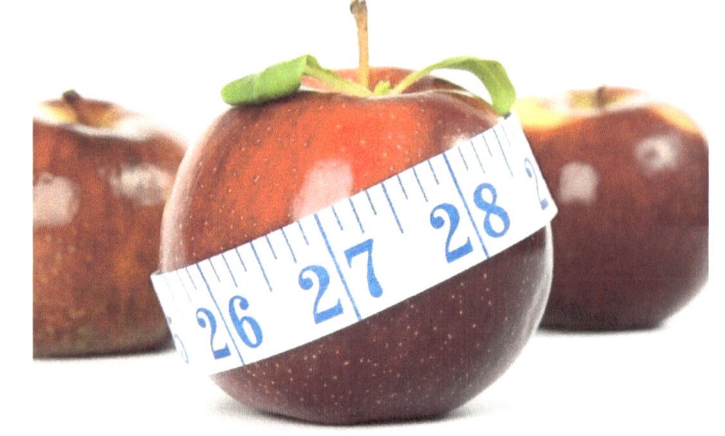

Body shame is a major psychological block that could be controlling your ability to lose weight. Whether you feel embarrassed about your general appearance, have shame about a specific aspect of your body, or have a traumatic event in your past that has shaped your body image, recognizing your body shame is the first step in overcoming it.

Share your body shame with someone you trust. If you want to make peace with your body and your feelings about food, you need to talk about it. If you do not want to share it with a friend or loved one, write about it in a journal or private blog.

Share your body shame stories with a professional or join an online support community. Talking about your body image issues can help you learn to deal with them and take steps toward overcoming the habits that have led to this point.

Distorted Positive Benefits

A huge psychological block to weight loss is the subconscious belief that you are getting more benefit from staying overweight than in losing the weight. This may sound crazy, but it makes sense for many, as losing weight presents a whole slew of changes in one's life.

It is also a challenge to lose weight and keep it off, so avoiding that challenge can be a payoff in itself and a way to avoid disappointment - again.

Your Turn: Consider carefully your *perceived* payoffs for staying overweight, then make a list and counter those with the health benefits of losing weight.

Belief In The Magic Diet

Believing that that "special magic diet" will save you is one of the most common psychological blocks to lasting weight loss. So, the merry go round goes like this, "oooh a new diet that promises fast results," you get on the diet, you lose 10 pounds and then you "get off" the diet and return to eating as you normally do. No lasting changes have been made, and so you gain the 10 pounds back or more. Then 3 months later, once again… "oooh a new diet that promises fast results," and here we go again….

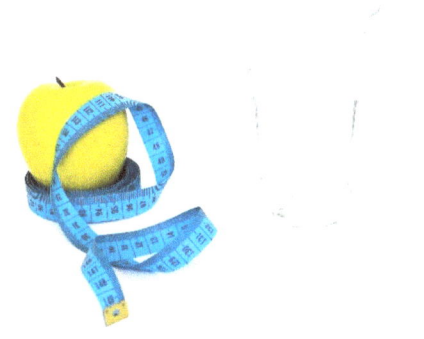

Sound familiar? How many times have you been down that road?

The truth is diets don't work. There is NO MAGIC DIET! The key to lasting weight loss is making profound lifestyle habit changes, which involve eating habits and also your mindset towards food.

Finding Joy In Food Beyond The Norm

This is another distorted thinking process where abnormally high levels of joy are connected to eating. Typically, this includes fatty and sugar-filled foods that actually affect the brain much like cocaine and heroin, causing instant and large floods of pleasure neurotransmitters to flood the brain.

Inability to Handle Discomfort

Fear of or lack of comfort with discomfort is another psychological block to weight loss. All change in life involves some level of discomfort, and a weight loss journey presents a lot. It is therefore very important to *"get comfortable with being uncomfortable"*. This is a life skill that can also help you many ways in life.

Practice is key, so spend 10 minutes each day in some type of discomfort. Sit out in the cold without a jacket, take ice cold showers, skip dinner, whatever makes you uncomfortable, just do it.

3 Key Mindset Shifts To
LOSE WEIGHT AND KEEP IT OFF

99% OF SUCCESSFUL WEIGHT LOSS IS PSYCHOLOGICAL

THINK LONG TERM HABITS NOT SHORT-TERM FIXES

If you look for quick fixes, you'll only get short term results. You need to stop thinking about losing weight quickly and start thinking about how to lose weight sustainably. Choose a plan you can follow for 5 or 10 years, permanently.

SUCCESS!!!

STOP BELIEVING IN THE "MAGIC DIET"

Believing that some "special magic diet" will save you is one of the most common psychological blocks to lasting weight loss. The key to lasting weight loss is making profound lifestyle habit changes, which involve eating habits along with your mindset, attitudes and thought process.

GET COMFORTABLE WITH DISCOMFORT

The weight loss journey presents many elements of discomfort. It is therefore very important to get comfortable with discomfort. This skill and change of mindset are key to weight loss and can also help you in other areas of your life.

Steps To Develop The Proper Weight Loss Mindset

Jay Nixon author of **The Overweight Mind** states that as little as 20% of weight-loss success is about diet and mechanics, the rest is mental. *"Getting a handle on [your] mindset is what leads to long-lasting results" (https://www.health.com/weight-loss/how-to-lose-weight-mindset).*

If you really want to lose weight and keep it off, then you must focus on changing your mindset first, not your diet. Changing your attitude about losing weight is the single biggest predictor of whether or not you will be successful. Your intention, inner resolve, and acceptance of yourself are all crucial for you to effectively change your behavior and your life for the long term.

Losing weight is not about fixing yourself. It's not about focusing on what's wrong with you or what you need to change. That is a negative mindset. Instead, **successful weight loss happens when you embrace the goal of lasting health, and set your mind in the proper ways, which will enable you to enjoy your life, live longer, and pursue the activities you want.**

You can learn new habits and develop new ways of thinking about food and eating. It just takes time and practice. It takes the right mindset and a focus on what is important. It takes getting your mind right so that your lifestyle choices can follow. Here are our top strategies for changing your mind so that you can change your life.

Prepare For Changes

- With weight loss and its journey come changes
- Dealing with challenges
- Changing habits
- Dealing with cravings
- Attention from others as your body changes
- A total change in lifestyle
- Saying goodbye to an older version of you
- And more...

Heartfelt Desire

The decision to lose weight may seem like one you make with your rational mind, but in reality, it is one you make with your heart. In your soul is where you get in touch with your deepest fears as well as your most heartfelt dreams, and in this lies the key to lifelong healthy habits.

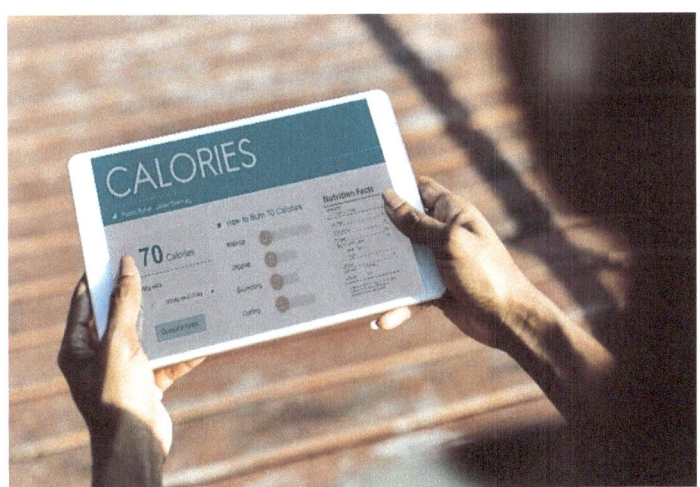

Motivation varies from person to person, it may be a desire to look good, or a more negative one that stems from fear, such as the threat of heart disease or Type 2 diabetes that results from overweight and obesity.

Your real motivation, what lies deep down, likely comes from a negative place, like fear. You may fear chronic disease or missing out on your favorite activities. You may be afraid that others will make fun of you or that you won't live as long as you would like.

While these are valid reasons to lose weight, you first must acknowledge that that is, indeed, where your motivation lies.

Think about what would happen if you did not make positive changes for your health. What are the positive consequences? If you want to make health a priority in your life, you must prioritize it for the right reasons. And focusing on the positive outcomes of these new habits is what will sustain over the long haul, not living in fear of what might happen if you fail. Keeping this positive motivation in the forefront of your mind and your decisions will enable you to be successful in your change efforts.

True lasting motivation always comes from your heart not from your head. A deep heartfelt desire goes a long way to lasting weight loss.

Make 2 Lists

1. Make a list of all the negative consequences of not losing weight
2. Make a list of all the positive consequences of losing weight

Make sure to be thoughtful and detailed in your lists as motivation is key in lasting success. Those who have solid motivation and keep it in the forefront of their mind for life, enjoy lasting weight loss success.

Learn From Your Mistakes

Instead of using your mistakes as a reason to berate yourself, learn from them. When you fail... and you will fail and have slips, learn from those, let them prop you up instead of tearing you down. Seek self-knowledge to avoid the same mistake in the future.

Learn From the Past

Instead of focusing on all the times you have tried and failed to lose weight, let your past be your guide. What can you learn from your past successes and failures that you can apply to your present situation? Don't beat yourself up about breaking promises to yourself in the past.

Instead, use those experiences as opportunities to gain self-knowledge, so that you don't have to repeat your mistakes again. We all fail from time to time; what is most important is that you learn from these missteps as you keep moving forward in life.

Make Your Goals Attainable

Often, that gung-ho feeling sets people up for failure. The first step toward getting healthy and staying that way is to start today by doing something. And the first inclination for many is to jump in with both feet, doing new things you have not done with your body in a long time (if ever).

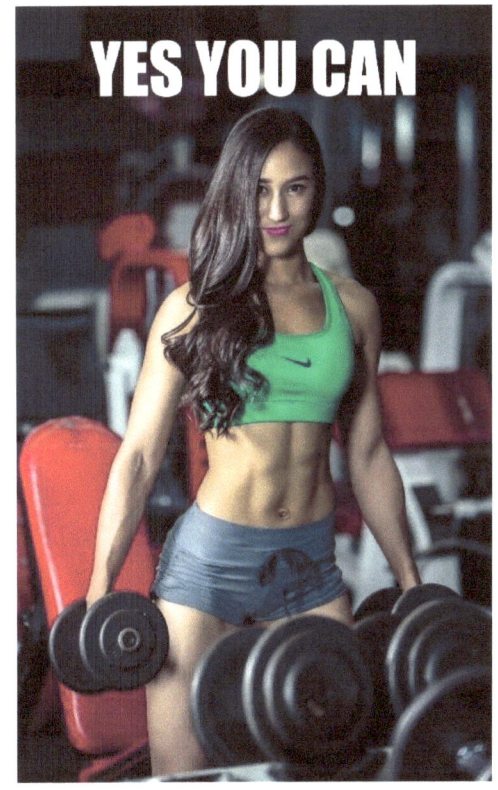

Instead of making it a goal to run for 30 minutes every day this week, start with a more attainable goal. Can you walk for 20 minutes at least three days this week? Meet this goal, then increase it incrementally, building up to your final aim.

Instead of focusing on big goals like losing 50 pounds, break it down into smaller goals of 10 or 5 pounds at a time. Those big goal numbers can be overwhelming and deter motivation to continue since it can take a long time to get there.

Another mindset shift that helps in this regard is instead of thinking I need to lose 50 pounds," think "Today, I will focus on changing bad habits, so I will eat a salad for lunch instead of a cheeseburger." One day at a time. One meal at a time if necessary.

By overloading yourself with expectations to make such drastic changes in your life all at once, you are setting yourself up for failure. Set real, attainable goals, and remember that each day is one of a million steps you will take toward your journey to improved health. And the only way you'll get there is by taking it one step at a time. *One day at a time. One minute at a time.*

Change Your Goals

Your goal should not be to lose weight. Your goal should instead be the more sustainable and important healthy habits you want to adopt in your life over the long haul. And your daily goals should be things you can accomplish each day to help make those new habits a reality. Instead of focusing on losing three pounds this week, instead, focus on eating at least five servings of fruits and vegetables every day for a week.

Instead of worrying about the scale, ask yourself if you are drinking enough water each day or getting enough sleep? Goals should be about your health, not about your weight. The scale does not define you. It informs you. Don't forget that.

Self-Control And Self-Discipline

Self-discipline isn't something you should just focus on when it comes to your food choices. It is something you should be practicing in all aspects of your life. Self-control is a skill, like any other in your life. The more you use it, the easier it becomes to use it and the stronger your willpower.

Self-control is a muscle that needs to be constantly strengthened for it to be stable and grow. **Every time you resist temptation, you develop more self-control.**

Resisting temptation is important in all aspects of your life if you want to be healthy, so learn to exercise your self-discipline in many ways, and you'll see how it pays off when it comes to your eating.

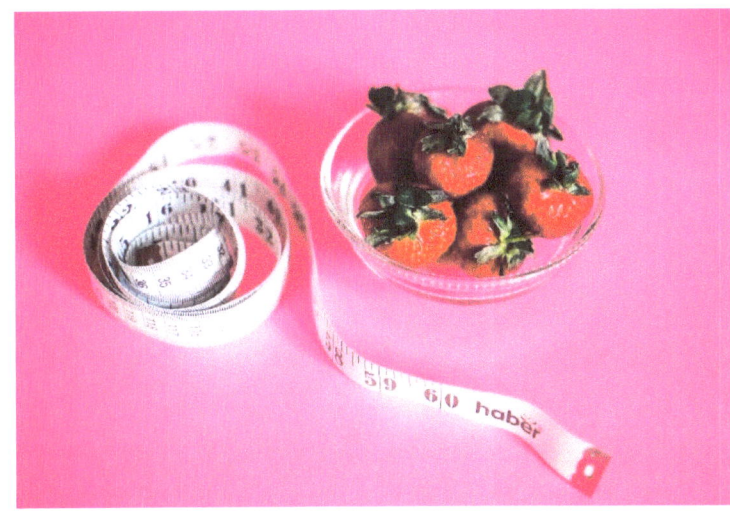

Ditch The Cant's

The word "can't" must be abolished from your vocabulary:

- I can't eat right
- I can't stand healthy food
- I can't exercise
- I can't lose weight
- I can't take the workouts
- I can't find time to eat right
- I can't cook healthy, so I" just keep eating out, whatever they serve

All those "cant's" bring you down, and it really is a matter of perception, and a false belief system, because in reality, you CAN do all those things. To start turning the "I cant's" to "I CAN'S," make a conscious effort to turn those "I can" statements into mantras. Change your mind from "I Can't" to "I CAN."

Be Grateful

Learning to be more grateful can actually improve your chances of successfully losing weight and living a healthier life. When you have more gratitude for the positive things in your life, you behave in more positive ways and feel better about the opportunities you have.

Being grateful also has been shown to reduce the presence of stress hormones in the body, which can lead to binge eating and other unhealthy habits. Start each day be acknowledging your gratitude to help make your healthy changes permanent.

Forgive Yourself and Others

Your regrets, grudges, and anger could be what's really weighing you down. Carrying around unresolved feelings, whether about yourself or other people, can keep you from staying positive and committing to the healthy changes you need to lose weight successfully. All those vivid emotions you feel during the day, including your suppressed road rage and your uncontrollable irritation at the barking dog next door, are coming from somewhere. And that place is where all your negative emotions go to hide. It's also where all your bad habits feed.

When you learn to forgive, you are much more likely to become healthier, feel less stressed, and remain focused on the positive goals you have set for yourself. Fixation of these negative emotions is a sign that you have not dealt with some of your feelings, which is crucial if you want to achieve health and wellness. Let it go, and you'll start to feel lighter.

Find Fulfillment In Life, Not Food

Eating preferences and patterns become much easier to change for good when you are getting what you want and need out of life in other ways. It's no coincidence that many people have successfully and permanently lost weight when they have changed jobs, pursued a dream, or removed themselves from an unhealthy relationship. Once you are happy in other areas of your life, you no longer need to find happiness in food.

You are not unhappy because you are fat. You are fat because you are unhappy. Knowing this means you can make the necessary changes you need to create more joy and spark more satisfaction in your life, which can help you make the kinds of healthy changes necessary to change your weight for good.

What do you want to do with your life? If you were entirely free to make any changes in your life that you wanted, what would you do? Look deeply into your heart to unearth your dreams, and you'll soon see that initiated positive changes in your life to make these dreams a reality will allow you to live the healthiest life you have ever imagined.

Reconsider Rewards

Becoming healthier is a way to take care of yourself. It's not a reward for good behavior or punishment for poor choices. Being healthy is the reward. In the same way, food should not be used as a reward, and exercise should not be considered a punishment. These are two things you do in order to care for yourself, which allows you to be the best person you can be.

According to registered dietitian Laura Cipullo, author of **Women's Health Body Clock Diet**, *"Keep in mind that making healthy choices is a way of practicing self-care, food is not a reward, and exercise is not a punishment. They are both ways of caring for your body and helping you feel your best. You deserve both."* *(https://health.usnews.com/wellness/articles/2016-09-19/10-ways-to-shift-your-mindset-for-better-weight-loss).*

Build a Community

Making significant changes in your life is difficult, especially when you are

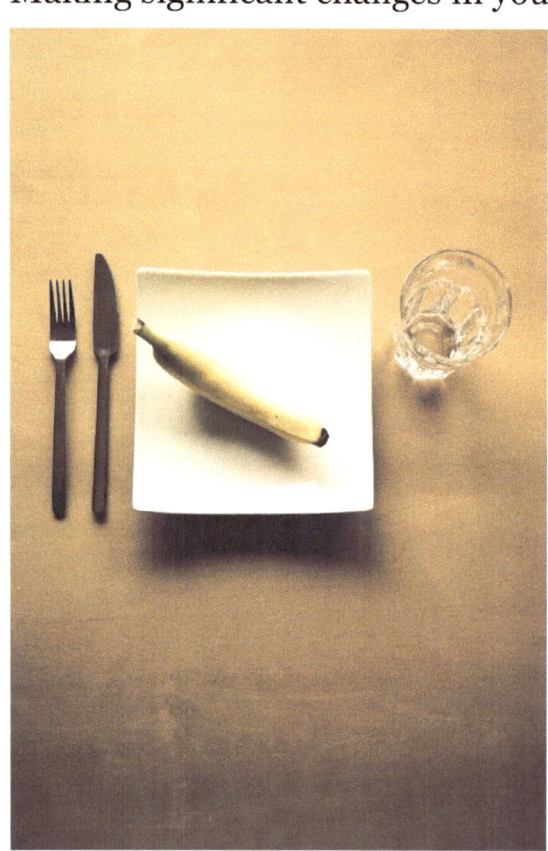

on your own. You alone are the only one who can make changes, but you can't make them alone. That's why it's always helpful to become part of a larger community that is dedicated to the same healthy lifestyle that you are. Your community can also focus on emotionally, mentally, and spiritually healthy habits that help to improve your overall wellbeing.

Those who have help from a supportive community are much more likely to achieve their goals. When you are trying to make changes alone, you can feel isolated and scared, which leads to anxiety and **depression**. These emotions are much more likely to derail your chances of success. So, stay connected if you want to remain successful.

If you don't like a face-to-face group, you can consider an online community. Or join a gym or become active in a club that engages in a particular activity you love. Whatever it is, find a way to connect with others.

Focus and Breathe

Establishing an intention in everything you do can help you to remain focused on your goals and what you believe is important. Start each day, each activity, each meal, and each workout with a moment of reflection. Take a few minutes to breathe deeply, to think about what you want to do and why you are doing it, and then begin.

Purposeful breathing and setting of intentions make it clear that you are choosing each of your behaviors. Things don't just happen to you; you make choices that make those things happen. This practice forces you to confront the many different options you make in a day to determine when and how you are opting for the healthiest possibilities you can.

Build Your Resilience

Being able to bounce back from obstacles and hardships means you have a capacity for resilience. Resilience involves patience, problem-solving, determination, and perseverance, which can combine to help you find ways to overcome challenges and start over after failures. Actionable goals you can do every day are better to focus on, and when you occasionally stumble at these, it's easier to bounce back, too.

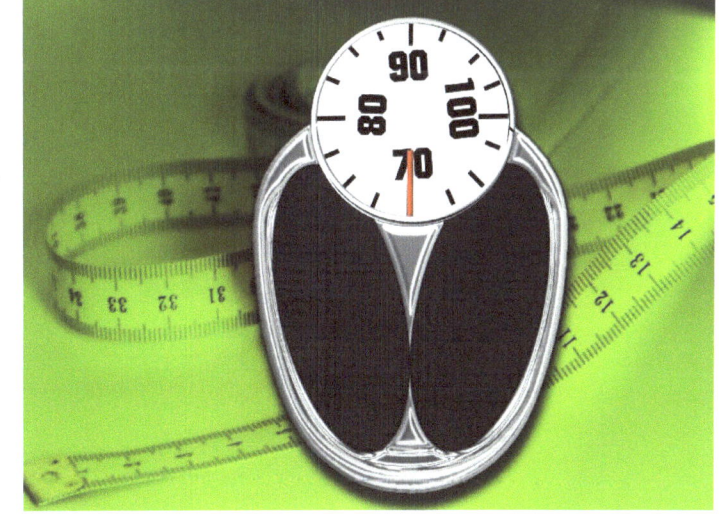

Being patient, a vital component of resilience is important to your weight loss journey. It takes time to safely and healthily lose weight, and you need to work every day at taking one tiny step closer to your goal. When we are so used to instant gratification, this can feel maddening. But patience helps you appreciate your hard work and acknowledge the value of what you are working toward, as well.

Break Up With Your Critic

We know how powerful that inner critic can be. We saw that in the first section. If that voice is controlling your life, then it's time to break up. Identify the negative thoughts that most often get you into trouble when it comes to your healthy eating choices and make a plan for how to change or stop them. When you hear that voice, stay "stop" out loud.

Say out loud the positive things you want to tell your critic that are reminders of why you are making these choices. Repeat this often, every time you hear the voice. Break the chain of the thought, and it is less likely to return. Repeat frequently, and you'll notice that, over time, that voice will disappear.

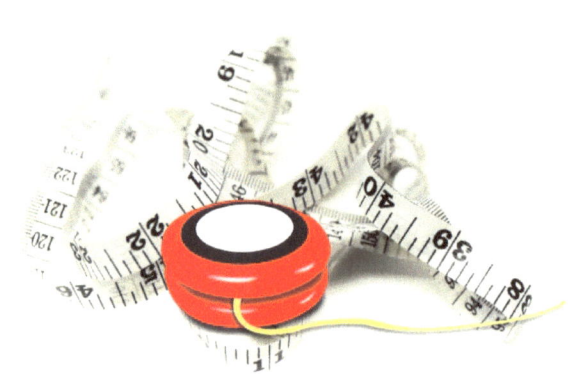

Become A Friend To Yourself

It is easy for many people to be very hard on themselves when it comes to their weight or appearance. The standards you hold yourself to are likely much stricter than any that others would even consider asking you to uphold. And you are probably much harder on yourself than you ever would be on someone else. Why the double standard?

Learn to treat yourself in the same way you would a friend struggling with the same issues. Treat yourself with compassion and respect if you want to learn to love and accept yourself.

Weight Loss Sabotage 101

There are a lot of issues that people dealing with weight control must face. There are obstacles like social stigma, cost or availability of quality food, and lack of proper dietary education, just to name a few. Some of these

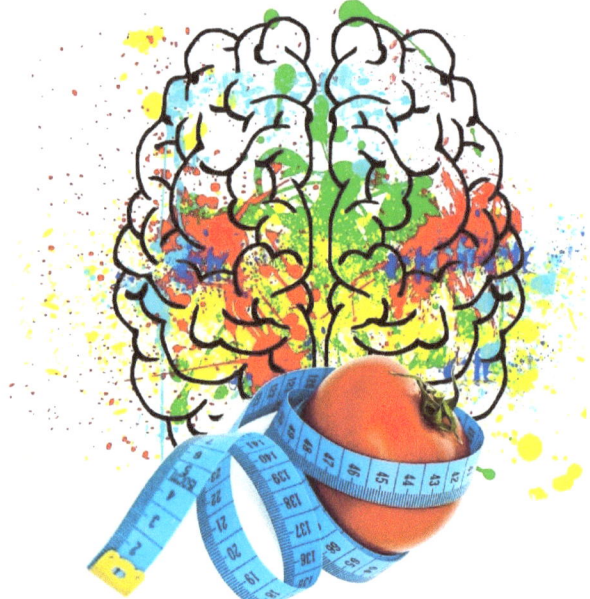

issues are self-imposed. But, how do you solve a problem that you're the cause of?

Playing the Victim

The first way that you can sabotage yourself is by allowing yourself to play the victim. Sustainable weight loss is hard, and it takes time. It can be easy to give up. Don't let yourself give up.

Similarly, many people rely on the idea of relapsing. If you are generally good with something, it can be all too easy to forgive yourself for the occasional slip-ups. So easy, in fact, that you might knowingly slip up and write it off as a "relapse."

Allowing yourself a little wiggle-room in your healthy eating plan can be a good idea for a number of reasons, but write that leniency into your plan so that you don't go overboard.

Trading Goods

Another way that you can sabotage your weight loss plan is by sacrificing one aspect to praise yourself for another. Sustainable weight loss is made up of physical activity and careful eating.

If you keep up on your exercise plan, it can be easy to justify more calories. Similarly, if you've been good with your diet it can be easy to forgive yourself for skipping a workout.

Both of these elements are important to lasting weight loss and favoring one instead of the other can be a dangerous path. If you only workout or only diet, your weight can continue to be a problem despite your perceived efforts and that can lead into the first problem that we talked about with playing the victim.

There is room for concern when it comes to exercise and calorie balance, especially on low-or-no-carb diets. This is a particular problem for people with **diabetes**. If this is something that you're genuinely worried about, talk about your concerns with your healthcare provider.

Not Working with Your Healthcare Resources

Not working with your healthcare provider can also be a way to self-sabotage your weight loss efforts. It's easy for people to talk about eating right and exercising more as if that were all you had to do. It's a good start but if weight is really a problem for you there are a lot of other things that you may need to balance. Your health care provider, or even healthcare team, can help you to navigate this space to get the most out of your weight loss plan and help ensure that you are staying safe on your weight loss journey.

Keeping up with your healthcare provider can help you to avoid annoying problems like plateaus as well as serious problems like over-exercise, under-nutrition, **low blood sugar**, and high blood pressure. If you aren't keeping up your relationship with your healthcare provider, you're not doing your best.

Not Working with Your Social Resources

Your healthcare team shouldn't be the only one that you are talking to. Keeping up with your friends and family can also be a valuable resource. Having a supportive community can make it easier for you to value your own achievements and to encourage you to keep working when those achievements seem few and far apart.

If you don't feel comfortable talking to your family and friends, try looking for community resources or groups of other people working together on weight loss. You are the most important person in your weight loss journey and if you are having problems on that journey, you could be the source of those problems. If this is the case, identify the role that you play and try to correct it. Losing weight will be much easier if you keep yourself on your toes and watch out for these and other common methods of weight loss sabotage.

Seeing A Mental Health Professional For Weight Control

You've tried everything to get the better of your weight, but have you tried talking to a psychologist or mental health professional? There are situations in which talking to a mental health professional may be helpful and appropriate but there are other situations in which it may not really make sense.

Maybe You Can Solve Your Own Problems

You are the first mental health expert that you can talk to. You may not have a degree or a lab coat, but no one knows you like you do, and no one is in a better condition or position to learn about you.

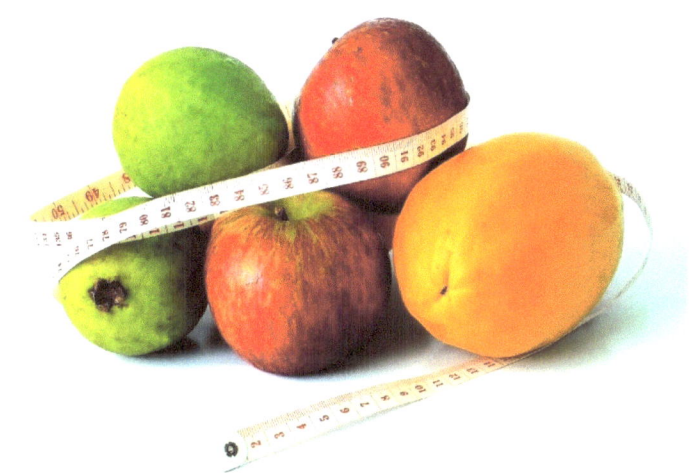

Many bad eating habits are just that – habits. One of the ways in which our minds creates habits is a way of simplifying common decisions. If you regularly do things in sequence, like hit a drive-through on the way home, it can be something that you feel like you must do. The problem is that you might not even recognize that this is happening.

Breaking these habits requires identifying them and you can do that by keeping a detailed diary. Keep a diary for a week or so and then go through it. Highlight bad food decisions and try to identify trends between them.

This can help you identify "triggers" that lead to bad decisions so that you can consciously try to avoid these triggers or interrupt the chain of events to break the habit.

Maybe Your Care Provider Can Help

Just like you shouldn't think of psychologists as the only mental health experts in terms of your weight control, you should be taking full advantage of your relationship with your primary care provider and dietician if you have access to one.

Some food habits and cravings have less to do with you as an individual and more to do with you as a human. The human body is hardwired to crave things that our ancient ancestors didn't have as much access to, like carbs, sugars, and fats.

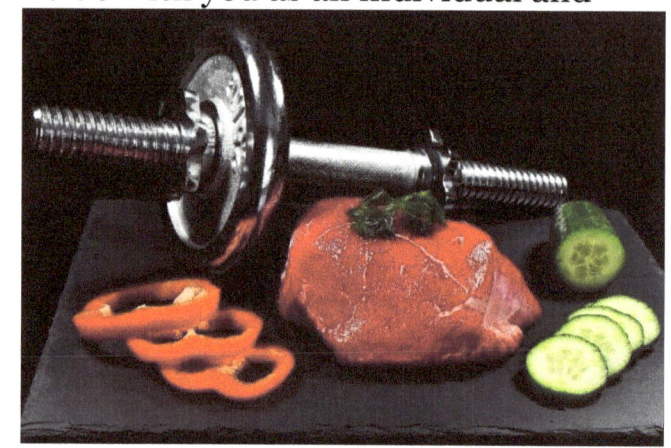

Similarly, some cravings are at least partially caused by messenger molecules in your body - specifically the stress hormone cortisol. It doesn't take a therapist or counselor to help you to navigate these relationships between you and your food.

Maybe You Need a Mental Health Expert

So, is it ever time to talk to a mental health professional about weight control? It can be.

It's true that you can learn about yourself and that doctors and dieticians may know more about "food psychology" than we tend to give them credit for. Sometimes the reasons that we can't control our own weight go deeper and a psychologist is called for.

There are issues that may need to be resolved with a mental professional in order to facilitate weight loss success, such as low self-esteem, body shame and other deep-seeded issues that can sabotage weight loss efforts.

Therapy can be helpful in changing your relationship with food. For many an unhealthy relationship with food is the core issue of a lack of weight loss success.

Behavior modification and Cognitive Behavioral Therapy (CBT) are known to work well for those struggling with weight loss.

Mental health professionals can be extremely useful for and are often required for those with food addiction, binging eating and emotional eating issues.

Some therapists use hypnosis to help patients lose weight.

Cortisol issues. Cortisol is a chemical released into our bodies in times of stress that controls what foods we crave and how our bodies use the nutrients in those foods. That means, if you have a high level of stress you may need a mental health professional to help you to manage stress – especially if that stress is because of a mood disorder like anxiety.

Similarly, people with depressive disorders may experience a lack of appetite and may not eat as much as they should. However, symptoms are different for everyone. Because depressive disorders often make it feel impossible to exercise, they can result in weight problems.

Working With A Mental Health Expert On Weight Control

One word about seeing a mental health professional about weight control: if your weight is aggravated by an underlying condition like depression or anxiety, a mental health expert will prioritize treating that condition.

Sometimes this involves medication and sometimes this medication can contribute to weight problems.

The good news is there are many treatment options for depression and anxiety so these may just be a temporary roadblock on your weight control journey rather than another permanent obstacle.

Further, some conditions like depression and anxiety can be worsened by body weight concerns and self-perception so while some mental health experts will focus on treating your mood disorder before your weight, others will see managing your weight as a way of managing your mood disorder. It all depends on your condition, your priorities, and your mental health provider.

Weight control problems don't always stem from mental health problems. However, sometimes a mental health condition is a cause of your weight problem. In this case, identifying the problem and working with the appropriate experts can be a life changing or even life-saving experience.

Lasting Weight Loss: Positive Reinforcement

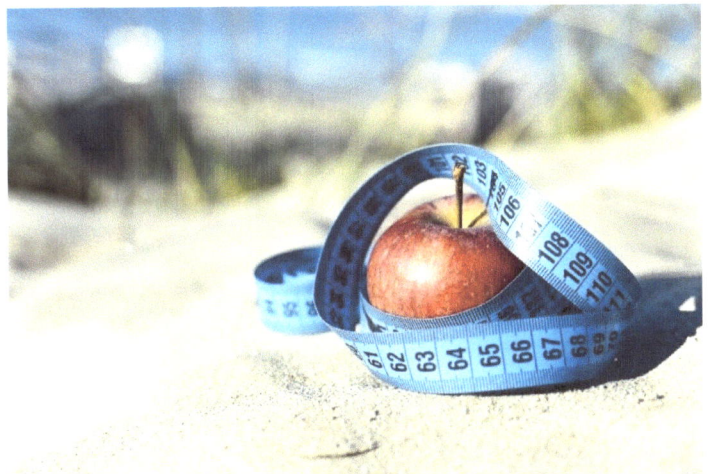

Temporary weight loss is one thing, but lasting and permanent weight loss is another. A lot of those popular diets and fads can lead to weight loss but it seldom lasts long. Sustainable, long-term weight loss required dedication and lots of time.

As a result, the resources that you need to achieve lasting weight loss are not only educational resources, but also workout gear, and good food.

While goals and a smart eating plan are needed, without psychological resources the chances of success fall drastically. One of these psychological resources is positive reinforcement. It can be a powerful tool if you know where it is and how to use it.

What Is Positive Reinforcement?

There is a lot of misconception about positive and negative reinforcement. Most people think that positive reinforcement means that if you do something good, you get something good – a reward, if you will. Similarly, they believe that "negative reinforcement" means that you do something good, but something bad happens to you – it's punishment. That's not exactly the case.

Positive and negative reinforcement are both forms of what is called "operant conditioning." Operant conditioning was developed in the early twentieth century by psychologists B.F. Skinner and Ivan Pavlov.

In operant conditioning, the individual comes to draw relationships between behaviors and apparent consequences.

1. Positive reinforcement means that when an individual does something encouraged, they receive something that they want.
2. Negative reinforcement means that when someone does something not encouraged, they no longer get something that they don't want.

How Reinforcement Is Used

Positive and negative reinforcement are most often used to train pets, but they're also used by parents, employers, corrections officers, and teachers to encourage specific behavior in the people that they are variously responsible for.

In the example of parents, positive reinforcement might be giving a child rewards for getting good grades while negative reinforcement might mean not requiring them to do chores at home if they get a job outside of the house.

In weight loss, positive reinforcement goes a long way to keeping you motivated and focused on your goals. When the payoffs are positive, people tend to continue that behavior.

Can You Practice Positive Reinforcement Yourself?

If you are trying to lose weight yourself and want to try positive reinforcement. How could you go about it? There are a number of ways.

Reward Yourself

- Compliment yourself and often on your milestones and small victories along the way, even the loss of 5 pounds is a big win

- Treat yourself to a movie, or a small gift after reaching your weight loss milestones
- Been eyeing a new outfit for a while? Go get it once you have lost some weight
- Look in the mirror each evening and congratulate yourself on another successful day
- Reward yourself for breaking a bad habit
- Recognize your achievements regularly, write yourself love notes for all you have accomplished

Note: Do not use food as a reward, this is not a positive reinforcement

Look for the natural rewards

With weight loss the natural rewards are great sources of positive reinforcement.

You go down a clothes size or two, note that and recognize it and celebrate it. Take those compliments from others seriously and with vigor.

Many experience big increases in energy after losing some weight, note that and celebrate it. Look for the other rewards you gain after losing some weight and recognize them too!

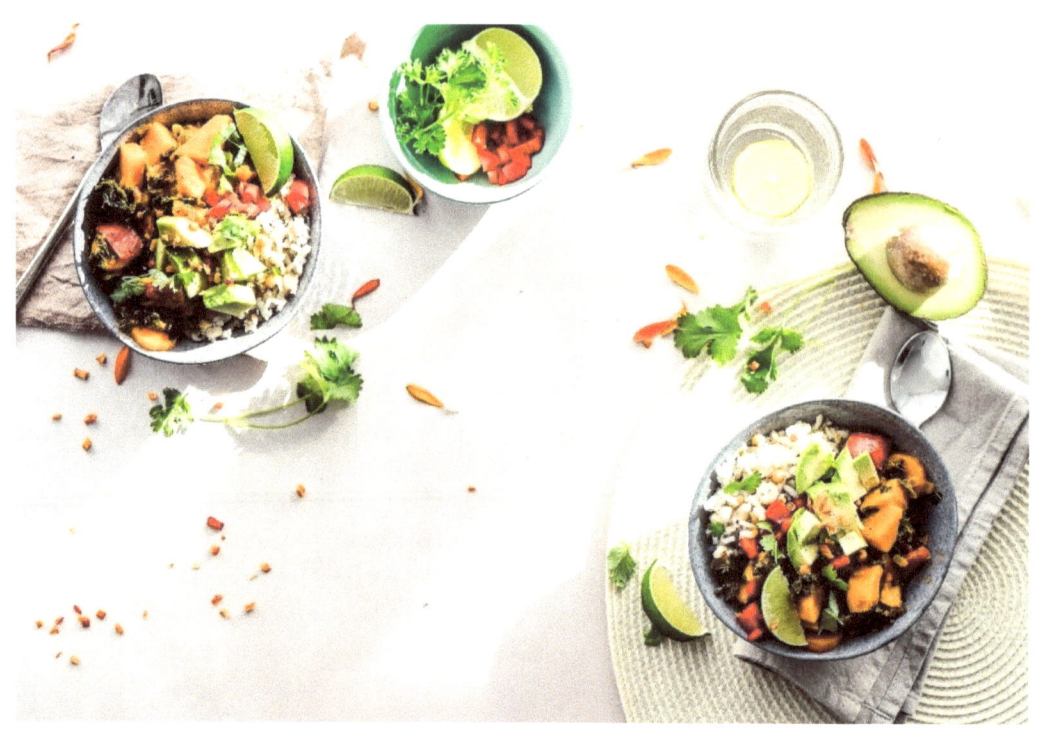

Your Turn: What's Stopping You?

What's stopping you from achieving your weight loss goals? This question and its answers are so important, take it seriously and take the time to consider the answers carefully. Be honest and thorough in your inventory. Doing this will help you overcome obstacles in your weight loss journey.

Exercise

Do you believe you can lose weight and keep it off?

What is stopping you? Or a better question to ask yourself yet is "What has stopped you in the past?"

Consider the psychological blocks to weight loss, which apply to you?

- Lack of Self-Awareness
- Self-Sabotage
- Weight Loss Sabotage
- Your Emotional Readiness
- Distorted Thinking
- Learning to feel satisfied with just being satisfied after a meal, and not stuffed
- Learning to identify real hunger versus a mental desire to eat (for other reasons)
- Being able to overcome cravings
- The ability to monitor food intake – which includes mindful eating and portion control
- Develop healthy coping skills for stress, and negative emotions
- Be comfortable with and accept that food restrictions and portion sizes are a natural part of a healthy weight

- Accept that lasting habit changes are needed for lasting weight loss and this means that healthy thinking must be maintained for life
- Poor Self-Esteem
- Emotional Distortion: Connecting Food To Feelings
- Living To Eat Versus Eating To Live
- Body Shame
- Distorted Positive Benefits
- Belief that staying overweight is more beneficial than losing weight
- Belief In The Magic Diet
- Finding Joy In Food Beyond The Norm
- Inability to Handle Discomfort

5 MENTAL CHALLENGES TO WEIGHT LOSS

PSYCHOLOGY IS 99% OF SUCCESSFUL WEIGHT LOSS

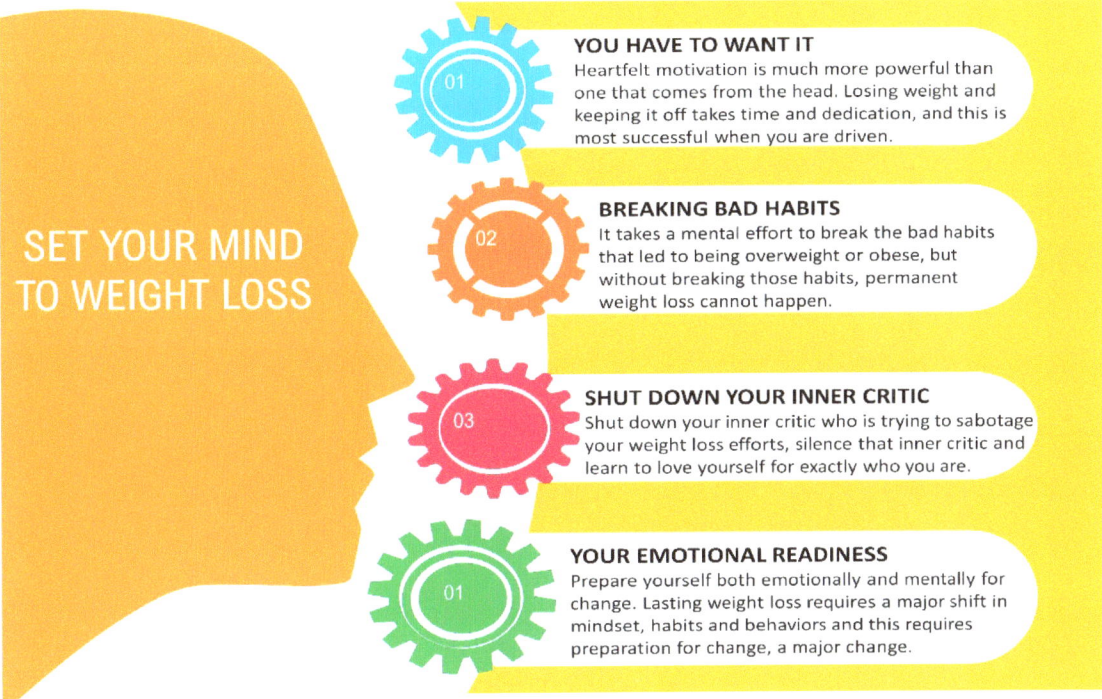

SET YOUR MIND TO WEIGHT LOSS

01 — YOU HAVE TO WANT IT
Heartfelt motivation is much more powerful than one that comes from the head. Losing weight and keeping it off takes time and dedication, and this is most successful when you are driven.

02 — BREAKING BAD HABITS
It takes a mental effort to break the bad habits that led to being overweight or obese, but without breaking those habits, permanent weight loss cannot happen.

03 — SHUT DOWN YOUR INNER CRITIC
Shut down your inner critic who is trying to sabotage your weight loss efforts, silence that inner critic and learn to love yourself for exactly who you are.

01 — YOUR EMOTIONAL READINESS
Prepare yourself both emotionally and mentally for change. Lasting weight loss requires a major shift in mindset, habits and behaviors and this requires preparation for change, a major change.

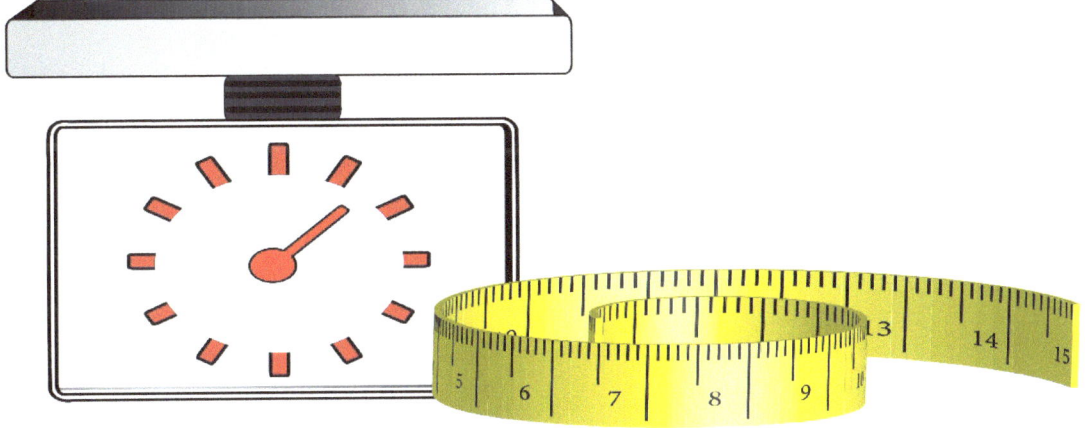

Final Thoughts

The next time you decide you need to lose weight, stop thinking about what's in your fridge and start first by thinking about what's on your mind. Your motivation and mindset are the keys to making lasting, healthy changes to your life, which is the only way you'll be able to successfully lose the weight you want and keep it off for good.

Change is hard, and it takes time. Gaining insight into your own mind and heart will help you understand your past mistakes, accept yourself, and learn how to create the healthy habits you will need to live the life that you want.

About the Author

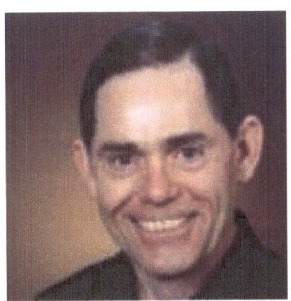

I have published numerous books on Amazon for Kindle, Draft2Digital. Lulu and other publishing platforms, both in electronic and POD formats.

While most of my books are on health and fitness in general, my topics of interest are leaning more toward aging baby boomers and the older population and the health and fitness issues they face.

Besides my own writing, I also ghostwrite ebooks, books, reports, articles, blogs and do Kindle conversions for clients on a variety of topics. Go to my website at http://ronknesswriting.com for more information or to submit a quote. For a complete list of my books, go to https://www.amazon.com/Ron-Kness/e/B0072M6PYO.

Today my wife and I are retired from our careers and live in San Tan Valley, AZ. I now write as a retirement business where you'll find me happily sitting in my office typing away on my laptop as I work on my next book or ghostwriting project . . . that is if we are not traveling on a cruise ship - our new-found mode of travel.

www.ingramcontent.com/pod-product-compliance
Lightning Source LLC
Chambersburg PA
CBHW060835290526
45792CB00006BB/1929